Becoming a
By Ashley Bergris

To my husband and son, for their never ending love and support.

TABLE OF CONTENTS

Preface

When my son was hospitalized for the first time, I searched high and low for resources that could help. It was almost impossible to find any, and there certainly didn't appear to be any books on the subject. I must admit I wasn't in a position to go searching at the time. Since then I've found online groups, blogs, and many other resources to help me through caring for my son. I hope to include the most important information here, in a format that gets straight to the point.

A "Medical Mom" is a mother of a child with medical difficulties. Typically these mothers have been through one or more hospital admissions. Their child may or may not have a diagnosis. At first they're frazzled and unsure, but over time they become staunch advocators for their children and their medical needs. My goal is to reach the frazzled and unsure beginners and expedite their development into the advocates their children need them to be. As you use this book feel free to skip around. I've made a sincere effort to enable each section to stand on its own. If you've stumbled over this book during one of many sleepless nights during your child's first admission, skip straight to the section

Surviving Admission and come back to the rest afterward.

The Starting Line

Everyone has to start somewhere. The journey to becoming a fully-fledged Medical Mama is no exception. Whether you have some medical knowledge already, or don't have a clue what any of the words the doctor is using mean, you're in the right place. I'm going to make sure you know the basics. By the time you're through, you'll know how to evaluate doctors, keep track of medical records, wrangle the insurance company, and survive hospital admission, whether it's a day or a month.

You can do this. I know it's overwhelming. The things the doctors say may not even be making sense right now. If you've already received a diagnosis, your head is still spinning trying to figure out what that means for you and your child. If you haven't, but your child is obviously struggling and no one knows why, you're not alone. There are a ton of women out there, just like you, which have no idea what's wrong with their child.

If you're a Medical Dad, let me apologize in advance. Most of the medical parents I know are mothers. Many fathers help, but the mothers frequently provide the majority of medical care to the child. If you are your child's primary medical caregiver, you're just as awesome as us moms! Please don't feel intimidated by the fact I refer to mothers throughout the text. It applies to dads too.

Your Medical Team

There are a lot of people that have come into your life due to your child's medical needs. Doctors, nurses, technicians, and more will interact with you on a regular basis to make your child as comfortable as possible. These people can be your best friends or your worst enemies, and the choice isn't always up to you which one they become. The most important thing to remember is to keep your child's best interest at heart. Sometimes the best healthcare providers have difficult, or even impossible personalities. They may, however, still be the best provider for your child. In some cases, it's worth managing your frustration with them closely to ensure your child receives the best care.

The intent of this chapter is to familiarize you with the parts of your child's medical team. If you've had significant health problems yourself, you may be familiar with this process already. If your biggest health concern is whether or not to actually go to the dentist every six months and the general practitioner once a year, then there's a lot to be gained in this section. There are different kinds of doctors, nurses, hospitals, and support staff. Knowing the difference will help you navigate the healthcare system.

Doctors

As a parent you're the one ultimately responsible for decisions about your child's care. However, doctors are the ones who will decide which choices you get to select from and advise you on which direction would be best to take. It is often the case, when your child has special needs, that all of the options are unpleasant ones. This can make doctors one of your more frustrating interactions on a day-to-day basis. You're not always going to agree with them. There is frequently no one to appeal to, because they're the authority on the matter. In cases where you believe their approach is genuinely incorrect, get a second opinion. If it's a relatively minor issue compared to more important concerns, consider saving your energy to fight the battles most important.

Medical professionals are just as diverse as the rest of us and you're not going to get on well with all of them. The important thing is what you do when things don't click. If you feel your child is getting appropriate medical care, then the answer is probably to grin and bear the situation. There are, however, exceptions to the rule. Doctors who you feel don't have your child's best interest at heart are never going to be a good fit for you and your child. Hopefully you pick this up early on, but if you don't you may need to change providers. This type of doctor is your worst enemy, and nothing you can do will make it better. If you're unsure of where to start looking for a doctor, generally an Internet search at google.com will yield results on any doctor in the United States. These links will then link you to other review sites and you can use whichever one is most comfortable for you. If you have private insurance, companies frequently provide lists of doctors participating in their network. Sometimes this information comes with a review similar to the ones you find on the public Internet. Don't hesitate to ask for a recommendation from your child's pediatrician, even if a referral isn't required. Pediatricians frequently have an excellent understanding of what each doctor can and can't do well. For a medically complex child, it's especially important to use a doctor willing to take the time and thoroughly review your child's case as well as be ready for any complications.

First and foremost is your pediatrician. Your child's pediatrician is the primary coordinator of their care in the majority of cases. All of the specialists you see are responsible for submitting a letter back to the pediatrician providing information about the visit. Depending on your type of insurance, your pediatrician may be the one to decide whether or not your insurance will cover a visit to a specialist. Even if this isn't the case, referrals from your pediatrician will go a long way toward finding specialists most appropriate for your child's needs. Every pediatrician has a lot of different specialists they work with. In my experience, they normally don't like to tell you specifically which doctor to see. However, your child has more complicated needs than others. If a specialist is more suited to the task of caring for a complex child, your pediatrician won't hesitate to tell you so.

Our first pediatrician was convinced that there wasn't anything wrong with our son. When I told her about his arching and crying while eating, she wouldn't believe that he had reflux. When he wouldn't gain weight she referred me over to her lactation consultant. Despite no improvement, she continued to have me work with the lactation consultant. The lactation consultant adamantly claimed he was getting enough volume and would spontaneously snap out of his weight gain issues. The scale clearly indicated otherwise.

By the time he was two months old, maybe even sooner, we were concerned about his survival, not just getting him back to a normal weight. At two and a half months we were referred to a pediatric gastroenterologist, but by then it was much too late. He stopped gaining weight entirely the weekend before our scheduled visit and we took him to the emergency room for what would become an approximately two week hospital stay. During the admission we found out about his milk allergy. His reflux was also officially diagnosed and properly medicated. We changed pediatricians before we left the hospital. Don't settle unless there really is no other option.

In addition to your pediatrician, your child is also likely to see specialists. These are doctors that have done additional study to focus in a certain field of medicine like gastroenterology, pulmonology, or immunology. Frequency of office visits varies significantly, but it's not uncommon to only see these specialists once every three to six months and follow-up with your pediatrician as needed between visits. They report back to your pediatrician about their findings and the pediatrician is responsible for understanding your child's overall picture of health. If for some reason a connection needs to be made between specialties the pediatrician will generally make it on their own. If you believe there should be a connection where there isn't, don't hesitate to bring it up with the pediatrician. Once you have a specialist in an area, your pediatrician becomes more hands-off in that realm of medicine. For example, if you have a gastroenterologist and your child has a feeding tube, you would call that specialist about concerns with how much you should be feeding your child by tube and what is "enough" by mouth to avoid having to supplement.

There will be times when you're concerned about the path you're taking with a specialist. You may disagree with it entirely, but that hasn't generally been my experience. My experience is that you and the specialist come up with a good plan, but it just doesn't seem to work. You keep trying and trying, and eventually you start to second guess whether or not the plan is the correct one. The specialist isn't going to change their plan, because it's their professional opinion. What do you do? In this case, a lot of specialists will recommend you get an independent second opinion. This is the ideal, and most professional way, to handle a situation where you really are concerned.

We went through this with gastroenterology. We were doing all the right things, but our son just wasn't gaining weight like he should be. Even though we trusted and had full faith in the specialist he was seeing, the concerns kept building and eventually we scheduled a second opinion with a gastroenterologist at another hospital with just as good of a gastroenterology department as the first. The medical opinion was the same, but the time wasn't wasted. It gave us a lot of peace of mind that we were doing everything we could and we just had to wait and see if any other symptoms presented themselves. We were informed some symptoms don't present themselves until after the child is a year old, so it was well within the realm of possibility additional insight would come later on. We've found this to be an accurate assessment.

What if the doctor doesn't suggest a second opinion? There are two possibilities. One, the doctor is receptive of the idea and just hasn't thought to mention it. In this case, you simply go and get the second opinion. The other is that the doctor is not receptive to you getting a second opinion. The latter, objecting to the second opinion, is unprofessional. I would not take my child back to any doctor that told me they didn't want me to get a second opinion. My reasoning behind this is, if they don't want you to get a second opinion, they must not think their approach will hold water when presented to their peers. If their approach can't withstand peer review, then it's not an approach I would recommend using with your child.

How do you tell the difference between a good or bad doctor? This can be difficult, because if you knew enough to know whether they were giving you the correct answer you wouldn't need them in the first place. Doctors are frequently the bearers of bad news, so it's almost impossible to judge them impartially. In order to decide whether or not staying with your current doctor is in your child's best interest, I recommend considering the following.

- Does the doctor care about your child? An easy way to find out is to ask, "Would you make the same recommendation if this were your son or daughter?" The doctor is always going to respond affirmatively. The key is *how* they answer. Watch their body language and listen to their tone. This way you can tell if the doctor sees your child as an individual, a case study, or a routine procedure.

- Does the doctor clearly convey what they believe is going on with your child, what they want to do, what they expect you to do, and why? If not, ask questions. Do you feel the doctor is rushing? Doctors are frequently behind, so it's normal for the visit to move along at a brisk pace. If the doctor is trying to leave before you've asked your questions or seems irritated by being questioned I would consider that concerning behavior. There are two primary examples of things that would cause me to immediately re-consider my choice in physician. First, being cut off. Second, if the doctor leaves the room without giving you a chance to ask questions and doesn't intend to return.

- Do you believe your input is considered important? You spend a significant amount more time with your child than the doctor. Your observations are valuable and provide significant insight into your child's medical condition. If you believe your child is in pain or their health is at risk and the doctor is telling you you're worrying for no reason, I would strongly suggest a second opinion. Even if you're wrong it will put your mind at ease and that's worth every minute of time spent.

- Are the doctor and staff accessible? Most of your questions are going to arise when the office isn't open. It's important to find out if the office has an emergency line, especially if your child is one of those cases where an occasional ER visit is expected.

Even with excellent doctors and specialists, you may run into disagreements from time to time. Ideally the professionals work these out amongst themselves and the disagreements stay within the care team without being exposed to the parent. However, if the professionals are unable to come to a consensus, then you have the right to decide upon an arbiter. In our case, I'm the arbiter. I talk to the relevant care providers and let them each make a plain English case as to why their approach is best and why they disagree with the other approaches. You can choose the best person for the job if you're not comfortable making this decision. Be aware that doctors are human and some have the same level of discomfort that you do about making the final decision when there's a disagreement. The ideal person to make the decision isn't the one with the most technical knowledge. It's the one most capable of listening to other's input and coming to a reasonable conclusion based on the provided information.

Why do I arbitrate? We have a multi-disciplinary team across three hospitals. The pediatrician has rights at one hospital, a few specialists have rights at another, and the rest are located at a third. It's a lot of pressure for any one doctor to stand up and make a decision, and while everyone takes leadership on his or her own specialty the potential for disagreement is still huge. We had a situation where our son was admitted for unexplained fever with no signs of illness, also known as fever of unknown origin. He went through a course of IV antibiotics and the fever died down so they sent us home, but it came back the next day. Our regular pediatrician was insistent she wanted our son re-admitted and given IV antibiotics until more tests could be run and the cause found. The hospital's pediatrician was insistent that our son should not be in the hospital, and that more IV antibiotics would only make a diagnosis more difficult and increase his risk of developing an antibiotic-resistant infection. With neither of the pediatricians willing to budge, I had to call both and try to understand what the fuss was all about. Once I understood the situation, we decided we wouldn't be admitting our son to the hospital. Was our pediatrician upset? Of course she was, and I don't blame her a bit. She truly believed her choice was the best one. We did find out later, his fevers are a new symptom and they come at go at their own convenience. This is why it's critical to educate yourself. Ask the doctors questions as much as possible. Some day you might be forced to decide which doctor's advice to follow and the more informed you are the better.

Nurses

There are two primary types of nurses you're going to be dealing with. The first is outpatient nurses. Outpatient nurses are normally a helping hand around an outpatient office. The second type is an inpatient nurse. You'll run into them at the hospital.

Outpatient Nurses

The outpatient office nurse can be a wonderful asset if you have a good relationship with them. They're frequently the one person that can advocate on your behalf if you know the doctor isn't going to agree with you. If they feel comfortable doing so, they can recommend a path forward and implement it with the doctor's approval. Doctors are so busy these days they rely heavily on their nurses to handle everything that is a medical concern but does not require their attention. There are some things you can do to keep a good relationship with the office's nurse.

- Don't hold back information or mislead the nurse. If something feels wrong the doctor may catch it causing the nurse to no longer trust you. Why would someone mislead a nurse? A parent might believe their child would be better off on a different medication, for example. In order to get the medication changed, they tell the nurse the current medication isn't working or vastly exaggerate the symptoms the child is experiencing.

- Leave brief and clear messages. If the nurse can figure out what you need before they call you'll simply get a call the problem has been fixed. It's a lot more difficult for them if they have to call you to understand the problem before working on it, but sometimes necessary depending on the issue.

- If you want to talk to the doctor directly, leave a message for the doctor. Sometimes the nurse will still contact you, but at least then they'll know you're looking for a discussion with the doctor or the doctor's answer. That way they don't put work into getting an answer you're not going to accept.

Inpatient Nurses

You'll encounter a lot of inpatient nurses once you're admitted to the hospital. They'll range wildly from being completely supportive to acting insufferably frustrating. When our son was admitted at three months old, the hospital observed us for a day and then took strict control of his feeding schedule and volume. After a few days of trial and error, they finally settled on a plan based on what an average baby of his size should need. We wouldn't find out until much later he needed more calories than average. The plan was to feed him every four hours. At three hours he would begin to fuss and whine. By four hours, he was crying inconsolably. One of the nurses that took care of us agreed he was getting hungry early and attempted to advocate on our behalf to give him more food. When that was unsuccessful, she made sure she brought his bottle at exactly four hours warmed and ready to go. For that 12-hour shift, it felt like we were being taken care of by an angel.

Inpatient nurses have something called orders. This is a set of instructions provided by the admitting physician or another doctor if needed which detail exactly what things the nurse is supposed to do for their patient. It includes medicine schedules and doses, any monitoring required, any dietary limitations, and many more things the doctor can specify at their convenience. These nurses call most of the shots with the exception of whatever is written in the orders.

There are two shifts, a day shift and a night shift. Each shift has a charge nurse that takes care of any problems that come up where the assigned nurse can't handle it on their own. This can be as routine as starting an IV on an unwilling child or as complex as teaching the nurse to use equipment they've never used before. The charge nurse is the person you talk to if you have difficulties with your nurse that can be resolved. For example, if you don't want your child woken while sleeping and the orders say nothing about waking the child or enforcing a strict schedule. You can ask the charge nurse not to have the child woken and the assigned nurse can be instructed not to wake the child, even if they disagree and want to wake them anyway.

At shift change, all of the nurses working go off and all of the fresh nurses come on at the same time. This is a hectic process, even though they do it every day. If possible, it's best not to schedule anything particularly time-sensitive around shift change. If it can't be avoided, make sure to remind the nurse that's leaving to tell the new nurse you'll need them immediately. If not reminded even important things might be delayed such as pain medicine or tube feedings.

Pediatric nurses generally work well together. The doctors are fairly hands-off. They write the orders and then leave it to the nurse to execute them. Most of the conflicts seem to be between nurses and parents. A good nurse is adept at avoiding these conflicts as well as doing their job. It's not uncommon to get a mediocre nurse that's either butting heads with you frequently or one that seems to have a difficult time doing their job. The pump is constantly alarming, the vitals don't stay attached, someone else has to come place the IV because they can't find a vein, etc. If your child requires a specific skill the assigned nurse doesn't have, it's fair to ask the charge nurse if someone else can do that particular task. The charge nurse will generally teach the assigned nurse to do it properly and that resolves the issue.

Is there a way to avoid conflicts with your child's nurse? Yes and no. If you disagree on the tasks that need done, it will need to be mediated by the admitting physician or a resident. Conflict isn't really avoidable in this case. If it's a relationship problem where you simply don't enjoy their company, then maintaining a polite and professional demeanor will solve the issue. You don't have to like the nurse, but you do have to deal with them for twelve hours. It's worth being cordial. This applies even if they aren't cordial. If your nurse is behaving rude enough it's making the admission miserable, definitely talk to the charge nurse and ask if there's anything they can do to help.

There may be times when you need to fire a nurse. It is possible, though not generally recommended. In order to fire a nurse, simply speak to the head nurse on the floor. You can request to speak to the head nurse either through the nurse you're having issues with or over the intercom. While you could ask a doctor or other staff member, nurse issues are best dealt with through the nurses themselves. If you are uncomfortable with this, the next best alternative is to request to speak with a patient advocate. Part of their job is to help you solve problems in the complex hospital environment. Your nurse can request the patient advocate stop by your room. If you're not comfortable asking your nurse, the nursing desk or one of the residents can help.

Consider beforehand the nurse replacing yours is going to be busy enough already without adding another patient. Be certain it's worth the trade-off.

If you can get along well with your child's nurse, they may even enjoy visiting. The best nurse experiences I've had are with nurses who've used our room as a safe haven from parents that won't leave them be. They look like they're working and they know if anything comes through that's a real concern someone will look in and grab them. If you need supplies, they just bring them when they come in next. They're frequently already present when your child needs their medicines. It's a win for both of you.

Having been through multiple admissions, I feel the need to tell you nurses are not as powerful as they would have you believe. There are things they do which are specifically designed to convince you they're the ones in charge.

- They direct you to do things, even if you already know to do them. This frequently starts off with a small command, but leads you into listening to them when they make larger requests.

- "The doctor said..." This one upsets me the most, because I've found in a small number of cases the doctor didn't say. In fact, the doctor hadn't even been consulted, much less asked a specific question and provided a specific answer. I knew this in one case because I had just gotten off the phone with the doctor telling me something different. The excuse was, "well that's what's in the orders. They need to be updated before I can do something else." This was also untrue. When the admitting physician came by the next day she informed me that the only thing in the orders is to do what Mom tells them.

- If you ask them to do something they don't want to do, and they can get away with it, they'll tell you they have to ask the doctor first. They'll then, "forget," to ask and say nothing, leaving you to believe the answer was no. Yes, it's possible they could've genuinely forgotten, but it happens a bit too frequently for me to give them the benefit of the doubt in all of the situations.

With these and other things, inpatient nurses can make your life extremely difficult if they want to. Generally, this isn't done out of malice. It's more so because they're doing what works best for them and not your child. The best inpatient nurses will ask you what you prefer instead of making the decision for you. Some hospitals have a technician that works with the nurse. If your nurse is difficult, you can rely upon them more as needed.

When I was in the hospital having my son, I couldn't walk for most of the day after giving birth. The nurse was likely too busy with other moms to make it in as frequently as I needed to go into the bathroom. The tech took excellent care of me and made sure I got to the bathroom within five minutes every time I needed to go. I don't recall seeing the nurse that day except for once when I first was placed on the floor and again at shift change.

If you're in a training hospital, and many of the good hospitals are training hospitals, you may be interacting with student nurses. I don't believe you need to deny a student nurse the chance to learn, but you do need to watch them closely. Some of them are more prepared than others to be in the hospital, and the ones that aren't prepared are dangerous.

During one of my son's admissions, the student nurse was supposed to prepare him for discharge which involved taking out his IV. She began to remove the IV without applying pressure to his hand, and he started to bleed all over his sheets. Worst of all, the instructor assumed this was such a simple task that she wasn't even watching! If you do decide to let the students into your room, watch them closely. Many of them have no hands on experience yet, and they really have little to no idea what they're doing.

Other Types of Nurses
You may also have a home care nurse if your child needs more care than you can be expected to provide. For instance, some children need 24-hour monitoring of vitals. These nurses tend to

become like family if they're with you a long time, but do not replace any member of the family. They simply become an additional caregiver along with Mom and Dad. Finally, some places have community nurses who can connect parents with community resources. These aren't available in all areas, including ours. Ask your pediatrician if this is something that might be available to you.

The Hospital

Your hospital is also part of your child's medical team. Which hospital you choose determines a significant amount about the care they will receive. Each hospital has things they do well and departments where they excel. If you have a diagnosis, simply research which hospital in your area is best in the applicable field. The best way to do this is to visit the hospital's website and read the doctor's biographies. They generally list a description of their experience and research topics they're interested in. Both of these things are a big clue whether or not they'll be interested in your child's case. If you're having a difficult time, your insurance company is familiar with providers in the area and can point you in the right direction. While I wouldn't use this as my first option, it's certainly valuable if you get stuck and don't know where else to look.

Sometimes, if you're very fortunate, you'll find a hospital and specialists in the field you need specifically interested in your child's condition. If you live in a remote area, however, your choices will be limited. You may not even have a children's hospital within reasonable driving distance. If this is the case, you'll need to consider moving. Weigh the cost of losing your support system against having your child treated by people unfamiliar with their needs. I would give this heavy consideration, especially if your child has a particularly rare condition. There are several major cities with multiple stellar hospitals. There is a significant amount of emotional distress hearing, "I don't know," from a specialist treating your child, which may offset the stress of having less support from family and long time friends.

Most hospitals have a quality website that lists information about each of their departments. This information generally includes what area their specialty is in as well as any specific conditions of interest. I don't endorse any particular site for finding hospital reviews. If you're unsure of where to start, generally an Internet search at google.com will yield results on any hospital in the United States. These links will then link you to other review sites and you can use whichever one is most comfortable for you. If you have private insurance, companies frequently provide lists of hospitals participating in their network. Sometimes this information comes with a review similar to the ones you find on the public Internet. Don't hesitate to ask for a recommendation from your child's pediatrician, even if a referral isn't required. Pediatricians frequently have an excellent understanding of which hospitals are best suited to treat children with special needs.

Without a diagnosis, things are a lot more complex. You'll need a qualified and competent medical team, not just an exceptional specialist. Since you don't know what the final diagnosis will be, it's sometimes impossible to find the exact right place for your child to be treated. In this case, you may need to consider working cross-hospital. You'll want to choose a primary hospital. Preferably it would be a children's hospital, as they're significantly better equipped for pediatric cases. Take what that hospital does best and use it to its fullest extent.

There are many reasons to have a second hospital caring for your child. Sometimes it's necessary because the first hospital doesn't do everything you need done. Other parents have a second hospital that's closer to home, and travel further to their preferred hospital when they feel they would be better suited to handle the problem. This is especially applicable if you don't have a children's hospital in your general vicinity. It's certainly worth driving the extra time, when possible, to be seen at a children's hospital. Hopefully, your child will never be admitted there. It's still important to be selective, however, because they will still be part of your medical team. They will run tests and provide significant input to your child's care in departments in which the primary hospital doesn't specialize. Information on how to manage communication between the two hospitals is provided in <u>Managing Your Child's Medical Records</u>.

One hospital resource you absolutely need to be aware of is what's called a Rapid Response Team (RRT). Not all hospitals have an RRT. I recommend choosing one that does as it gives you someone to call who has to respond quickly. This is especially helpful if you don't believe your child's current providers are taking his condition seriously. The RRT's responsibility is to arrive on short notice with a whole new team of doctors and nurses that perform a quick evaluation of your child. The purpose of this is to prevent death in patients whose condition is deteriorating rapidly. If you believe at any point that the care your child is receiving in a hospital is placing your child at risk of death, don't hesitate to request an RRT. The fact that you want a Pediatric RRT will be obvious if you're in a children's hospital or on a pediatric floor. If neither of those is true, don't hesitate to request a Pediatric RRT directly. That way you get the pediatric team if your hospital has one.

The Rest of Your Medical Team

Aside from the previously mentioned big three, there are a lot of other healthcare providers that will come in and out of your life.

Children with complex medical problems can reasonably end up with multiple therapists and a social worker to help connect the family with additional resources. It's not unusual to also have a home nurse visiting after your initial discharge, and a medical supply company delivering things your child will need but you can't just run to the store and pick up.

Therapists are fairly similar both inpatient and outpatient. What they do varies greatly depending on your child's needs. They are advocates for your child. Think about them like a sports coach. They're not there to do the job, but they do everything they need to in order to get your child where they need to be to do the job themselves. They're generally receptive to input and flexible in my experience. If you find that their methods don't appear to be working, consider getting a second opinion. Like doctors, there isn't a way to appeal their decision if their mind is made up.

Having a social worker has a certain stigma to it due to Child Protective Services (CPS). Their purpose when assisting at your request is to help find resources to better care for your family as well as your child's needs. This may include things like support groups, childcare providers that take children with medical needs, or information on government resources you wouldn't otherwise know about unless you were searching for them. For example, each state in the U.S. has an early intervention program where the school system provides certain services, such as therapy, which will come to your home and work with your child at no cost to you. I would love to tell you the name, but the names are frequently completely different from state to state. Early intervention is the generic name and can be used to find the program's name through the state government's website or through an Internet search. You must be referred and qualification for the program depends upon whether or not your child is behind in more than one development area.

Home nurses are very similar to inpatient nurses, except they come to your house. At a minimum, their role includes making sure you have all the resources at home you need to provide adequate care for your child. This generally includes making sure your medical supply company has received the supply order and that the supplies have been delivered. In some cases where the child is struggling significantly, the nurse will visit on a weekly basis to monitor the child and prevent re-admission. Your medical supply company is either going to be easy to work with, or a royal pain in the neck. The reason behind this is you need your supplies in a certain timeframe and if they're delayed you may not be able to provide your child the care that they need. Some will make the system fairly straightforward, predicting your needs and reading off a list of items they expect you'll need as soon as you call. Others put you on hold, sometimes for multiple hours, to even place the order in the first place. When the order actually arrives it may or may not be correct. If you have a medical supply company that's impossible to work with, talk to your insurance company about switching. The insurance company always has their preferred contract, but they may have another supplier they cover if a parent is having a particularly difficult time.

Understanding Your Child's Medical Information

Some health professionals are better than others are communicating complex medical concepts. It also varies from field to field whether concepts can be communicated in simple terms. It's fairly common for a significant amount of meaning to be lost when the information is put in plain terms. For this reason, and others, it's important to ask questions about anything that's unclear. Any questions you had before going into the appointment need to be written down prior. This will facilitate being actively engaged and able to ask questions about any new topics that come up during the visit.

It's particularly important to ask what a medical term means if it's used during the visit and you haven't had time to look it up beforehand. It's already difficult to absorb what's being said and there's no need to add additional challenges. There is no such thing as a stupid question when it comes to your child's health. You are your child's advocate, and it's important you work as hard as you can to understand what's going on in order to make the correct decisions. Some ideas for handing visits include:

- Write your questions down ahead of time.

- Keep logs of how your child is doing, and remember to bring them to every appointment. This can help you show the doctor trends in your child's behavior. For example, if your child eats well in the morning but refuses food entirely at night, logging their food intake will not only prove the point, but will show the true severity of the problem.

- Take notes of the doctor's response and check your list of questions to make sure they've all been answered. If you would rather record the visit most doctors will be fine with it, but ask first.

- Review the doctor's orders before you leave. Do you understand what they mean? Do you have all of the necessary equipment and materials to follow the instructions?

- After the visit, make sure any labs or follow-up diagnostic tests are performed promptly. If they must be delayed, leave a message for the doctor and let them know.

- Call after the results are expected. As much as I would love to tell you, "No news is good news," in this case you want to confirm. A faxing error, a misplaced paper, or a busy doctor can all delay or prevent you from finding out critical information.

***

In the information age, when we need to educate ourselves about something we are accustom to Googling the information. You will have many questions about your child's condition, so it's natural to want to search for information online. However, please, do not attempt to diagnose your child by searching for symptoms on the Internet. If you manage to convince yourself by Internet search the doctors are wrong and you know exactly what's wrong with your child, you'll end up fighting them tooth and nail over treatments which would be beneficial.

There are an unreasonably large number of websites that claim to be experts on medical topics. People run some of these sites with absolutely no medical training whatsoever. What's worse, they frequently end up cited by respected data aggregation sites and look much more authoritative than they would if you visited the site itself. Whenever you see a site or use a data aggregation site, look for references. If there are no references, don't use the site. Medical data is thoroughly cited and even a doctor who has studied many years in an area would still site the appropriate resources when making a claim. **Avoid message boards entirely.** It's impossible for the average person to know the true identity of the person that's posting. Just because they claim to be a doctor, nurse, or other expert doesn't make it true.

If you do get a diagnosis, it's always a good idea to look it up online and understand as much as you can about the condition. Looking up a definition of a diagnosis given by a doctor is significantly different than trying to diagnose your child through Internet search. It's an excellent idea to be informed on the details once the doctors have pinned down what's wrong with your child. If it looks worse than your doctor described, don't panic. There are frequently differing severities in a diagnosis and your child's may be on the milder side. This guideline goes for medical terms as well. If you're reading through something related to your child's care and find a word you don't recognize, please look it up. Continuing to learn about medical terms related to your child's care and information about their condition is critical to providing the best care possible. There's no such thing as knowing too much in this situation. You're a health care provider now yourself, with one very special patient that's well looked after day and night.

Managing Your Child's Medical Records

Medical records' accuracy is ultimately the responsibility of the parent or guardian of the child. Any time you sign, you're attesting to that document's correctness. You're also responsible for ensuring any information that must be transferred from one provider to another is sent and received. Medical records are difficult to manage, even between two doctors. When you have multiple doctors across multiple hospitals it's extremely easy to miss sending information to all the places it needs to go. Even if you make the request and sign all of the appropriate forms, the records themselves may never be received. Between calling to make the request, signing forms, calling to ensure the information has been sent, and calling to confirm the records were received, it can be a full time job in and of itself. Despite the difficulty, it's worth all the effort required.

These records have a huge impact on the quality of care your child receives. When you have a child with special needs, the impact is even larger. Whether or not the doctor has the records from your child's other providers, they'll still try to help.

Unfortunately, if they don't have the background on your child's condition it's generally impossible to fully convey all the necessary information in one visit. Additionally, there are things in the office visit reports and test results that may never have been conveyed to you. The information may not have seemed relevant at the time the report was written, but if combined with recent developments it might provide significant insight.

Why do I have to take care of this? Can't the provider request the records? The answer is both yes and no. There's a law called HIPAA (Health Insurance Portability and Accountability Act) that, among many other things, provides rules for management of medical records. A provider cannot request records on your behalf unless you're an established patient with a medical records release form completed. If you're seeing a new doctor or specialist, you will have to submit a medical records release form to the sending office. This way you can provide the records in advance. If you don't send the records in advance, they won't be able to ask for them until after your first office visit. You'll need to inform the provider where your records are, and what information is available to request. You'll still need to provide a signed medical records release form, but you won't have to send it yourself.

The easiest way to handle this is to have the new provider's office e-mail or fax you a records release form. Ask them to mark what specific records they want on the form prior to sending it to you. That way, you know you're requesting the correct things. For example, if you request an MRI record, often what is sent will be just a report on the MRI and not the images. If the specialist would like to review the images, they need to specifically request the CD be provided in addition to the report. Once the form is completed, send it to the provider that has the information. The records release form provided by the new office will have all the information for the exchange and, typically, no further intervention is required. You'll want to call and confirm the information has been received at least a week before the visit to the new provider, just in case the records request was misplaced.

Can I have copies too? Yes, you can, for a fee. It doesn't cost anything to transfer records from provider to provider. Occasionally, if you're making a small request, an office will send you something without charging. More often than not you'll need to pay for any records you'd like to have. Whether or not you request records for yourself is entirely up to you. If you choose not to, it's still important to review your child's information from time to time for accuracy. You have the right to ask to see your child's medical file. It's important to do this from time to time, but it's critical if you think something incorrect has been entered. For example, your discharge papers from a recent admission list a condition you don't believe your child has. Don't sign them, ask to have it explained to you why the diagnosis was made or have the discharge paperwork corrected. Errors may turn into problems down the road if not addressed.

My child has a lot of specialists at different hospitals. How do I keep them all up to date? It's difficult at times, but it's possible. The important thing to remember is each hospital has its own software system, which holds its patient information. That means, if you saw a doctor at one hospital, every other doctor at that hospital can see his office visit report as soon as its submitted. So, really, all you have to do is make sure you keep the information up to date at both hospitals. You don't need to send all the information to each provider.

When Things Just Don't Add Up

You have a connection with your child, and it's even deeper and stronger than your commitment to them as a caregiver. When children have medical needs, their primary caregiver develops deep instincts in relation to their care. These instincts are subconscious. At some point, if it hasn't happened already, you're going to know for a fact something is wrong with your child but have no tangible proof. How others around you respond is completely unpredictable. They may be supportive and they may not, but that doesn't change that your instincts are very real and need to be taken seriously.

Supportive responses may be things like, "I don't think anything is wrong, but I'll give you a ride to the hospital." It's unlikely that someone will just point-blank believe you because your child may look completely fine to an outside observer. Un-supportive responses vary from, "you're such a worrywart," to, "you just want something to be wrong with your child." I wish I could tell you the latter statement is uncommon, but it's not. Be especially cautious of people who make those types of statements to you or your partner. These are the people most likely to claim there's nothing wrong with your child and you're making your child sick. Their perception is truly that you're making up everything you're telling them. People in your life who hold the opinion that you can't be trusted to care for your child cannot be as active in you and your child's life as you would like them to be. Whether or not you can continue to have a relationship with them at all depends upon the actions they take in response to what they believe is happening. We'll cover this further in The Dangers of Unsupportive People.

When our son first came under the care of a pediatric gastroenterologist (GI), they calculated his intake based on his weight and wrote a prescription for the exact amount of formula we were told to feed him. The first week of any increase in formula he was always less fussy and tired, but soon returned to fussing, whining, and crying prior to his feedings. It was especially common for him to wake up in the middle of the night and refuse to go back to sleep.

I advocated endlessly on his behalf to have his formula increased. Time after time I was told it wasn't possible he was hungry and they were already giving him more calories than he needed. When he reached a year old and transitioned to toddler formula, they had us visit with a nutritionist. I begged her to increase the amount of formula, and did my best to explain that he just needs more calories. She agreed, and was able to document his higher calorie need. He now sleeps mostly through the night and has enough energy to play during the day. Depending what your instincts tell you to do, even you may not take them seriously. For example, your child is warm to the touch but their temperature is in the normal range. They're sleeping a lot, but they also stayed up late last night. Something inside you knows they're getting sick, but the information in front of you just doesn't lead to that conclusion. In this case there's no reason to do anything, the illness will show itself in time and will probably be treated symptomatically anyway. Unfortunately, sometimes it's not that easy.

There may be a day when, for whatever reason, you get the feeling that something's off. It's persistent and doesn't go away. You can't pinpoint what it is, but it feels urgent that you call the pediatrician. *Do you put it off? What would you even tell them?* Don't put it off. Call the pediatrician, even if it makes no logical sense. When you're talking to them, tell them what you've seen and heard your child do that day. You can even say directly, "I've just felt like something's not right with him today." Our pediatrician takes that sentence seriously, and yours will too.

I hope it never happens, but one day you may feel the need to rush your child to the Emergency Room. Something's not right, and they're just not themselves. It doesn't seem to be getting better, the fever's not going down, and your instincts are screaming at you. Place an emergency call to your pediatrician and tell them what's going on. They can call ahead and let the Emergency Room (ER) know you're coming and will be happy to do so if they agree the situation is an emergency. Call an ambulance, or load your child into the car and head to the ER immediately if instructed to do so. The phone call from your

Pediatrician to the ER will *significantly* reduce the amount of time it takes for your child to be seen. You're a Medical Mom now and you have to trust your gut.

Surviving Admission

If your child has special needs, chances are they'll be admitted to the hospital at some point and you'll probably be with them. I've yet to meet someone that wanted to be in a hospital. There are so many things that become significantly more difficult after you're admitted. I'm going to tell you about the big ones and you'll find other little tips and tricks as you go along. Let's begin with our basic needs, food & water, shelter, and sleep.

Food & Water: Hospital food is always a struggle. No matter how good of a job the cafeteria staff does, it's still cafeteria food and cafeteria food just isn't that great. You know who is even sicker of the cafeteria food than you are? Nurses! Your nurse can hook you up with a large list of all the places that will deliver to the floor in a pinch. If there are places on the hospital campus, and your kid is really cute, sometimes you can schmooze free babysitting. A five-minute trip to Subway feels like you've just been released from your own personal hell after about day three. Water is usually easy. There's an ice machine and water fountain on every floor in every hospital ever. You just have to find out where it's located. If you're there for an extended stay you might want to drink something besides water. There's a good chance the hospital staff has a fridge somewhere you can keep sodas, tea, etc. in.

Shelter: Usually when you talk about shelter you talk about going into a place from outside. In this case, it's more of an occasional escape from your assigned room. Some rooms are bigger than others. If you're in a children's hospital there's probably a playroom somewhere. Haven't been told about it yet? That's because your nurse is too busy thinking about the many different patients she has to remember that you only just got there need to be told things, like how to play with your kid and not let him roll around on the floor of his hospital room. The lava game is only fun for about four hours, and after that it gets old. Depending on how your child is doing health-wise you might be able to swing an exit pass. Ask your nurse if you can have one. Generally it's OK unless your child is quarantined or requires continuous monitoring. I'm sure if you know how good that five minute trip to Subway feels, you can imagine how being able to take your child somewhere that isn't constantly sanitized would be really nice. If you can't leave the floor, you have my deepest sympathies. It usually doesn't last but, if its longer term, talk to your nurse. There's generally television and other forms of entertainment available, which might not be immediately obvious.

Sleep: Lastly, and most importantly, is sleep. While you're in the hospital, nurses or technicians will come by to do something called vitals. They are not sleep friendly. It generally involves taking their temperature, blood pressure, blood oxygen level, and pulse rate. If you're fortunate enough to have a child that can sleep through vitals and a nurse that can do them gently enough to make that possible, you're extremely lucky. For the rest of us, just ask the nurse to hold off until morning. It won't hurt to ask, because if the doctor thinks the vitals are important he will communicate that in the orders and they'll just say no. An experienced nurse can make a reasonably accurate educated guess whether or not a child has a fever based on their heart and respiratory rate. If you can get the hospital staff to leave you alone so your child can sleep, you've solved the first part of the problem.

If only your child was the only person in the room that needed to sleep! Depending on the room, you may have a couch or a chair. I tend to think of hospital couches as being closer in relation to outside benches than actual couches. Depending on the state of the, "couch," it might actually be more comfortable to sleep on a firm bench! Unfortunately that's not an option, so you have to improvise. Hospitals frequently have an overabundance of pillows. Feel free to make a nest. Anyone who displays even a hint toward judging you has either never slept on a hospital couch, or has forgotten what it feels like. I prefer the chair myself. They're generally padded and if you're really lucky the reclining function actually works. I curl up in a nice little ball between the armrests with a couple pillows and I'm as good as I'm going to get for the night.

Once you've figured all that out, then there's showering and clean clothes. Ideally you have someone that can switch off with you for a few hours and let you shower at home and do a load of laundry. If not, just do the best you can. Showering in the room, while unpleasant, beats smelling like you've been in the hospital for a month after two or three days. For laundry, you can generally find a kind soul out of all of your friends and family members that will come by once a week and toss your clothes in the wash, dry them, and bring them back.

Depending on your home situation, you may have to deal with a significantly more complex set of issues. Your other children will need a place to stay until things can go back to normal. Ideally they can stay home with Dad, but that's not always possible. When it is possible, try to keep them in their normal environment. Even if you have to swap in an unfamiliar caregiver, the familiarity of home will reduce the pain of disrupting their routines. It will also minimize the pain of getting to and from school and being away from friends. If you can't do any of these things, don't feel guilty! You're doing your best in a difficult situation, and they'll adjust just fine to whatever environment they're placed in if necessary.

Even with the kids settled, it still may not be practical for you to stay at the hospital the entire admission. You may need to work to keep your job. As the admission wears on, there may be things you need to take care of at home that your husband simply cannot do. Your other children may need you for one reason or another and are not always permitted by the hospital to visit with you and their sibling. If you can, swap with your partner. Otherwise, as with your other children, find someone as familiar as possible to keep watch over your child. If the only thing pulling you home is your other child (or children), consider using a video calling application like Skype or FaceTime. That way they can see and talk with you, and you won't have to leave the bedside.

It's not advisable under any circumstances to leave your child in the hospital alone, though it is sometimes impossible to avoid doing so. A responsible adult, ideally you or another legal guardian, needs to be there to make sure your child is cared for and supervised. You may need to make some difficult adjustments to your living situation to guarantee someone can always be with your child. If you need to leave your child with someone who isn't one of their legal guardians, make sure they can reach a legal guardian quickly in case important decisions need to be made about your child's care. Unfortunately, children cannot advocate for themself effectively. Even with strict instructions, the staff will not necessarily follow your guidelines once you step out the door.

Medical Insurance

Dealing with medical insurance companies is difficult.

Sometimes things that are supposed to be paid for aren't, and things that you wouldn't expect to be covered actually are. Sometimes things are covered, but only under certain conditions. For example, many insurance companies cover formula if it's a specialty formula that's medically necessary. However, this is only true if you have your child's GI doctor write a prescription and send it to the medical supply company.

In the United States, insurance is not provided to everyone. My experience is with private insurance through an employer. If you need insurance and don't have it, contact your state for assistance. They'll be able to tell you if you qualify for any subsidies or government programs that pay medical bills in whole or in part. Even getting catastrophic coverage with a high deductible can be a significant savings when you have a child that needs frequent medical care.

If you have private insurance like I do you've probably discovered they can be intimidating. If they give you an answer about whether or not something is covered it feels final. When you get the bills in the mail from providers it's easy to assume they've billed the insurance correctly and what they're asking for is what you owe them. Unfortunately, even though both of those things appear to be generally true, they're not always true. The first step to increasing your awareness is to begin reading your benefit statements. Each time a provider bills your insurance a benefit statement is issued to you. These statements tell you how much the insurance told the provider they were permitted to bill, how much the insurance paid, and how much you owe the provider. If the provider is in-network, meaning they take your insurance and agree to abide by the terms offered by your insurance company, then you are only responsible for what is listed in that statement. It's against their agreement with the insurance company for them to bill you any additional costs for that service.

As you look through the statements you may find errors. Some things that look like errors are a problem and some aren't. It's important to contact the insurance company first to find out everything that's in the statement. Sometimes a billing code's short description will sound like it can't possibly be right, but when you hear the long description from the customer service representative with your company a small subset of that billing code does in fact apply to the service you received. If you still believe you're being billed incorrectly after you talk to the insurance company, you'll need to discuss it with the provider. Every doctor's office I've worked with so far has had at least one person that handles medical billing day in and day out. They'll help you figure out what's going on and explain why they think they're billing correctly, or they'll change the code.

In rare cases you may end up in a situation where things still don't seem right. The next step is to open a case with the insurance company. One of the insurance company's customer service representatives will be assigned to resolve the case and, theoretically, the insurance company and provider's medical biller will get together and figure out a resolution. Sometimes the case gets resolved in your favor, sometimes not. The important thing is to make sure you're getting the benefits promised to you by your insurance company. If they're not covering something they should, it's absolutely your right to push back. The only catch is, if you use an out-of-network provider, they may not help you resolve the issue. For this reason, we stay in network the vast majority of the time.

***

If you haven't reviewed the benefits provided by your insurance plan lately, now would be a good time to take a look. Now that you have a child with medical needs, medical care is going to be a lot higher of an expense for your family than it ever was before. There are many different types of plans, and which one is right for you may have changed since your child's illness. There are a few important terms you need to know to make this decision.

1. Deductible – With a deductible, you pay 100% of the cost of your medical care until you reach a certain dollar amount. Once you reach that dollar amount, co-insurance kicks in and begins to give you a hand. Many plans don't have a deductible so don't panic if you can't find it in the plan information.

2. Co-Insurance – The insurance company pays a significant amount of the cost of your care, but not all. You may pay a percentage or a co-pay depending on the type of plan you choose.

3. Out of Pocket Maximum – At a certain point you may pay enough on your own behalf that you hit your out of pocket maximum for the year. Once you hit your out of pocket maximum, the insurance company covers 100% of your medical bills.

Unfortunately, some of you will hit your maximum out of pocket every year. In order to figure out what plan is best for you, combine the out of pocket maximum with your insurance premiums through the course of the year. That amount is how you'll compare insurance plans. If you can, put aside money during the part of the year where you've met your out of pocket maximum. That way, the full brunt of the medical bills won't be quite as painful the following year. If you don't hit your max out of pocket every year the decision is a little more complex and it's harder to provide guidance. You'll need to take inventory of all the costs you expect to have and figure out which plan covers them best. It's not easy, but its well worth the time spent and may save you a significant amount of money in the long term.

Diagnosis

At some point in your journey your child may receive an official diagnosis. Not all Medical Moms get a diagnosis, and your child isn't struggling any less if there isn't a name for what's wrong. You will never forget the day you hear your child's diagnosis for the first time. I can't tell you how it will feel, because everyone reacts differently. I can tell you, you can't possibly overreact. There is no reaction too great for finding out that your child has a chronic or severe medical condition. Even a less severe diagnosis, where the prognosis is very good, still may not necessarily give you relief.

If you're too emotional to discuss the details with the doctor, then tell them so. They will understand, and will be willing and able to come back later after you've had time to absorb the information. Don't feel the need to be the messenger. If your spouse needs called then it's OK to ask the doctor to call them. You don't have all the information right away and you can't be expected to absorb it right now anyway. It might be helpful if they hear it from someone who can answer their questions in case they're in a place, emotionally, that they can think of questions to ask.

Leading up to a diagnosis is an emotionally exhausting journey that may take months, or even years. Some parents want a diagnosis and some don't. Some parents can't decide whether they want a diagnosis or not. There is no guarantee you'll get a diagnosis and there are many children out there who are undiagnosed either because the condition is so rare it's not yet documented or they just haven't found the right doctor to connect all of the pieces together. The journey is worth making because many conditions are treatable, even some rare ones. It's painful to put your child through every test under the sun, so even the doctors won't do a battery of tests all at once. They'll run a set that seem promising, and if nothing helpful comes back they'll run another set. Once the other likely possibilities are ruled out, you may end up referred to genetics where they'll search for an underlying genetic diagnosis, which explains all of your child's symptoms. If that comes back inconclusive, then they may re-visit with you every year to see if medical advances have provided any insight and treat your child's medical problems symptomatically.

There are good and bad things about having a diagnosis if you do get one. The best part is you'll be able to predict or prevent future health problems that generally develop with the condition. The worst is potentially finding some bad things that aren't preventable. Even in patients with a poor outlook, it's very possible to beat the odds and do better than expected. For example, there are a significant number of children out there whose parents are told they would never walk and they learned despite the doctors' expectations.

It's completely normal to struggle with either getting a diagnosis or finding out your child is not currently diagnosable with available medical technology and research. You may not expect it, but you may experience a strong sense of loss when you do get the information. You'll go through grief just as you would with any other loss, and it will eventually get better.

The Dangers of Unsupportive People

Every parent of a special needs child I know of has had to deal with someone who wasn't supportive of his or her family's situation. For the most part this will be an annoyance, and I hope in your case it never goes any further than that. Unfortunately, some people's experiences aren't so mild and I need to share information with you about how to avoid ending up in a similar predicament. I wouldn't wish any of these things on my worst enemy. I strongly recommend, to a degree I can't properly convey in writing, to limit or remove anyone who is egregiously unsupportive from your life.

Everyone's definition of what it means to be supportive is at least a little different, and some are substantially different. When you ask for support from someone, what he or she gives may not feel like support at all. In fact, it might even be more harm than help. To me providing support means to listen, help with chores, and entertain the child when possible. I find it unsupportive for anyone to attempt to alter our routine or to criticize me to others. In order to avoid misunderstandings, communication is key. If you ask for help from someone you do generally need to accept whatever help they're willing to provide. However, many people will ask what they can do to help and you can then tell them a specific thing.

There are degrees of this, and I'm going to try to progress through from easiest to the worst. That way, if you have someone who is simply being a nuisance you can skip the rest of this section. Some people will downplay how much work and effort your child is and aren't kind about assisting when they do come to lend a hand. I find people like this to be more stressful than helpful no matter what you ask them to do, and would recommend leaving them to their own devices and not asking for their assistance.

There are times when you'll have someone that is helpful, but they'll constantly be making "suggestions." Depending on the topic of these suggestions, they may also be more stressful than helpful. For instance, if they're trying to tell you how to fold laundry then you can simply let them take care of it instead. However, if they're trying to tell you to change your child's medical care, doctors, or insist upon knowing medical details, be wary. In this case, instead of helping they're trying to step into the role of primary caregiver for your child. If they also insist upon going to doctors appointments, seeing medical records, reviewing logs, and begin calling your child's doctors, then something needs to be done. You, as the parents, have the right and responsibility to make medical decisions for your child. No one else's opinion belongs on the table unless you truly want it to be there.

The former two examples are generally well meaning. Unfortunately, that's not always the case. Sometimes the prying into medical records and calling doctors to get information is more malicious. There can be many reasons for this. They might believe you're lying about your child's medical condition. They may not think there's anything wrong with your child at all and are trying to prove they're right. Either way, someone who doesn't believe your child is actually sick certainly has no business being involved in the medical care aspect of your child's life. Some people won't admit to this, so if you suspect it to be the case I would go ahead and cut them off anyway. Realistically your child's medical information is no one's business but the parents' anyway.

Finally, there are people who take it one step further and attempt to have your child taken away from you. This would come in the form of a call to a physician, nurse, or directly to Child Protective Services, (CPS) with whatever accusations they feel are appropriate. If you suspect someone might be preparing to report you to CPS, or are encouraging one of your child's health professionals to report you to CPS, they're nothing but poison. There's no good that can come from continuing to keep them involved in your life because any involvement they have is going to become more ammunition for them to report you to CPS or your child's doctors.

My general recommendation is to exclude anyone from your life that behaves inappropriately or suspiciously. Any attempts to access your child's medical information, contact your child's doctors, or instruct you on the medical care of your child need to be taken very seriously. If someone doesn't meet your definition of supportive and your child is medically complex, there's really no way to have a healthy relationship with that person.

Medically complex and special needs children are too involved to spend time and energy on people that don't contribute love and positive energy to your environment.

Your Evolving Identity

There are a lot of women that lose their identity while taking care of their sick child. What do I mean by this? Having a child changes everyone to some degree, but it tends not to alter your overall life goals. Having a child that's medically complex or has special needs will temporarily change your overall life goals if you allow it to. Caring for a child with special needs can easily take every bit of time and energy you have to spare, leaving little for other things. If not used wisely, what little time and energy you do have left will disappear as if it never existed at all.

Your original life goals don't go away, they simply get pushed to the back of your mind. If you let this happen and completely lose track of them, you may find they're impossible to get back on track later. For example, if it's a career goal you might not be able to start over and obtain the same level of position and salary you would have if you had worked part time instead of quitting.

At some point your child may not need as much of your time and attention as they do now. It's important to spend some time maintaining your sense of self. The best way I've found to do this is to keep the activities I enjoy as much as possible, and scale back the commitment as needed. For example, I publish to my blog several times a week. If, for any reason, I can't take the time and sit down to write I might only blog once a week or even skip a week. If you continue doing the things you love, you'll have more energy to spend taking care of your child. It benefits both of you for mom to have a break sometimes.

If you can't, for whatever reason, stay involved with the things you enjoyed before, then explore some of the things you wanted to do but never took the time to try. I completely understand if you think this sounds silly, but please, try it anyway. Discovering you have a passion for painting, photography, writing, or another quiet activity that's easy to stop on a moments notice will change your life.

For those of you who see themselves as professional women, I'm keenly aware of what you might be going through. When I was pregnant with my son I fully intended to take six weeks off and then rush right back to work. In my profession, it's horrible for your career to take time off of work. Technology moves way too fast to keep up if you're not doing the job continuously. The profession is male dominated, making it abnormal to take even minimal time off for having a child. The amount of pain I went through in college to get my degree made the career extremely important to me. I also have a talent for it, which is practically a requirement to getting the degree. I knew staying home was going to end my professional life in its current form. I put off the decision as long as I could. First, I asked for six weeks. Then I extended it to eight. It wasn't until I extended to twelve weeks that I realized I needed to make a decision.

Going back to work wasn't meant to be, and I don't regret my choice to stay with my son in the least. Over the course of the last year I've come to accept my new identity, and I like the new me. I would be lying if I said it was an easy journey. It was difficult and there were a lot of pitfalls. There were times when I would have done anything to go back to work, but my son was too important to me to leave in someone else's care while he was struggling with his health. I carry no regrets.

You will make it through this. If your former identity no longer fits, you'll find a new one. It sounds overwhelming now, but time will help. Your child's condition may improve. You may find a sitter that can handle whatever medical needs your son or daughter has. The future holds a lot of possibilities. As long as you keep trying to maintain your identity, you'll be able to keep moving forward. If the time comes when it needs to change, you'll know. You're the only one that can make that decision, and you'll be ready when you need to be.

Working

The unfortunate reality for a lot of families is that they can't afford for either parent not to work. There are some ways to juggle this if you have the right skillset. Some professions can work from home and still provide significant contributions, even if they attended their meetings in their pajamas, on mute, with their child giggling in the background. Some workplaces have a good enough childcare program that you really could leave your child with them and check in every few hours without feeling guilty. The ability to provide emergency help on a moment's notice is priceless when your child has health problems.

If you can, consider going part time. Then, if you need to leave your child with a sitter they're not with the sitter all day long. Maybe you can work four hours every day instead of eight. That way the caregiver only has to handle some of your child's medical needs and medicines. Maybe you can avoid the caregiver handling medical needs or medicines at all, depending on the times worked.

If you do work full time, don't let anyone make you feel bad about it or guilty. Even if you do it by choice, you'll leave your child with a fully competent caregiver and they'll be just fine. The most important thing is for you to be happy with the choice you make. If you're happy with what you're doing, your child is going to be happy too.

We decided it was best for us for me to go part time. The way we handled it is that I work evenings, after my husband gets home, and Saturdays. My husband works the regular nine to five schedule Monday through Friday. He gets to spend quality time with our son and I get to get out of the house during the week without the baby in tow. You can't go wrong doing what works best for you and your family.

Taking Care of Yourself and Your Spouse

Having a child with medical needs causes a lot of things to be put by the wayside. When time starts to become scarce it's normal for caregivers to cut back on taking care of themselves. Their own health and relationships suffer and, while this may work out in the short term, it may have significant negative long-term effects. When it comes to the health care of you and your spouse, it's important to continue seeing whatever providers you need to see to stay healthy. If you do need to spend less time with these visits, please reduce them instead of eliminating them entirely. There is a significant difference between seeing a specialist once every year instead of once every six months and not seeing them until you can find the time. Finding the time may take several years, depending on your child's condition.

When people think of health care, they tend to focus towards the physical aspects. Maybe you do a yearly check-up. You might go in if you have an infection or an illness that you just can't seem to shake. This is an important part of your care and I will at no point minimize how important it is to take care of yourself physically. There is, however, another aspect of care that's often ignored: mental health. For some it's because of stigma. For others, they don't know resources exist to help. There are professionals out there who specialize in helping with stress, relationships, anxiety, depression, etc. You don't need to have all of these things to go see them. Simply being under a lot of stress is plenty of reason to see someone who can help you talk through your troubles and come up with solutions.

If you've never needed help with your emotional health before, start with a therapist. Since you have children, a family therapist would be a good choice. They specialize in dealing with issues that impact entire families. Your child's medical condition certainly qualifies as a problem that affects all of you. If speaking with the therapist doesn't seem to be helping enough that you feel like you're managing well day-to-day, consider seeing a psychologist. Psychologists have the ability and training to prescribe medications. Some people do go to the psychologist first, and while I don't recommend that approach I wouldn't say that it's wrong either.

I feel fine right now, is there anything I should do? It's definitely a good idea to find a good therapist before you're in the middle of needing one desperately. It's common not to feel comfortable with the first therapist you work with. You may need to see a few different therapists to find one that works well for you. It's completely reasonable to establish a relationship with a therapist and then call them when you really need them, or see them infrequently (e.g., once a month).

***

I wish everyone had a good support network. Unfortunately, it's not the case. Even more frustrating, there are families that start out with a good support network and lose it for reasons outside their control. Enlisting the help of a family therapist is essential if your support network is either not present, or thins significantly over the course of your child's illness. You need an independent third party to talk to when you're not comfortable talking to someone involved in the situation. Family therapists also have the ability to work with groups of people (e.g., mom and dad) and resolve conflicts when things come up that can't be resolved without outside help.

It's never too late to get help, and there are people out there that want to help you be at your best to better support your child. If the situation seems completely overwhelming, or you're simply too busy to find someone to assist you, that's when you need help the most. Your primary care doctor or insurance company can always recommend a provider for you to see, even if you don't have time to find them yourself.

Made in the USA
Charleston, SC
23 October 2015